Health Matters

Exercise and Your Health

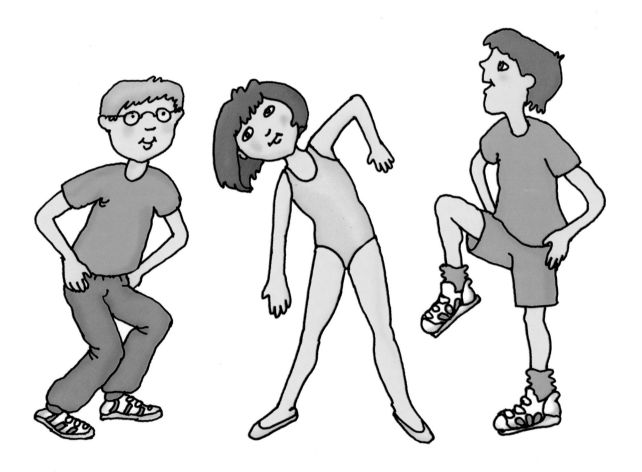

by Jillian Powell

RAINTREE
STECK-VAUGHN
PUBLISHERS
The Steck-Vaughn Company

Austin, Texas

Titles in the series

Drugs and Your Health
Exercise and Your Health
Food and Your Health
Hygiene and Your Health

Published by Raintree Steck-Vaughn Publishers,
an imprint of Steck-Vaughn Company

Library of Congress Cataloging-in-Publication Data
Powell, Jillian.
Exercise and Your Health / Jillian Powell.
    p.   cm.—(Health Matters)
    Includes bibliographical references and index.
    Summary: Describes various exercises for strength, stamina, and suppleness and the benefits derived from them.
    ISBN 0-8172-4927-3
    1. Exercise—Juvenile literature.
    2. Health—Juvenile literature.
    [1. Exercise. 2. Health.]
    I. Title. II. Series: Health matters.
    RA781.P63 1998
    613.7'1—dc21   97-19065

Printed in Italy. Bound in the United States.
1 2 3 4 5 6 7 8 9 0 02 01 00 99 98

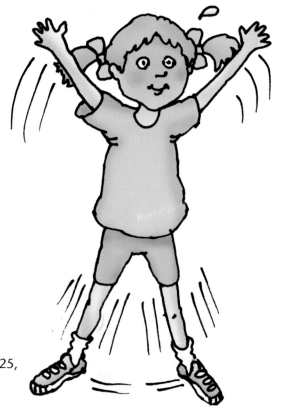

Picture acknowledgments
Action Plus 18, 28, 29; Tony Stone 7, 23; Wayland Picture Library/(Chris Fairclough) 4, 6, 11, 14 (top), 17, 19, 22, 24, 25, 26. All other photographs Wayland Picture Library.

Contents

Exercise Is Good for You

Your body is like an amazing machine. It needs to be used to keep it working well.

Using your muscles makes them stronger.

Exercise keeps your body strong and fit. Fitness means having the energy to work and play and do all the things you want to do easily. Your body cannot store fitness. You need to exercise regularly to stay fit.

Your heart and lungs are muscles. They need exercise to keep them working well and to help you fight off illness and disease.

While you are still growing, exercise helps your body make strong bones.

Exercise makes you feel and look better. It keeps your body a healthy weight by using energy from the food you eat.

When you exercise, your body makes chemicals called endorphins. They go to your brain and make you feel good.

Exercise helps you relax and sleep better. It is like a magic tonic for your body, but you need to exercise every day.

You keep fit by making healthy choices about what you do and what you eat.

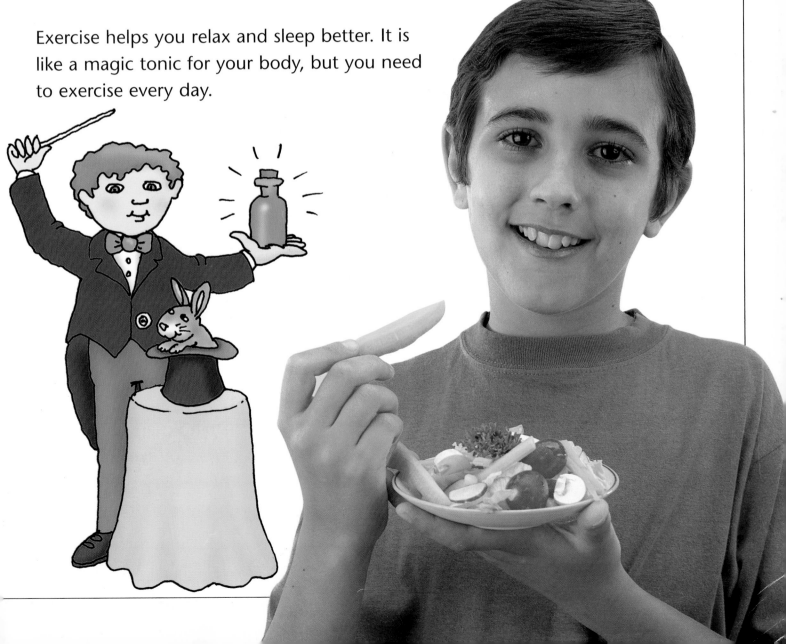

Strength, Stamina, and Suppleness

You need to do different kinds of exercise to be really fit. Exercises for strength make your muscles stronger so you can work different parts of your body without feeling weak.

Exercises for stamina make your heart and lungs stronger and help your blood flow easily around your body. Stamina is the ability to exercise for longer without getting tired or out of breath.

Exercises for suppleness help your muscles and joints move freely so you can bend, stretch, twist, and turn without feeling stiff or sore.

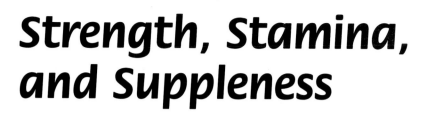

Doing many different types of exercises will help every part of your body work better.

How fast is a fit human?

A snail moves at .03 mi. (.05 km) per hour.

A human sprinter can run at 27 mi. (43.37 km) per hour.

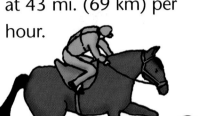

A racehorse can gallop at 43 mi. (69 km) per hour.

A cheetah can run at 62 mi. (100 km) per hour.

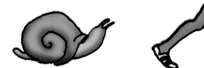

If you get out of breath running upstairs, you need to improve your stamina.

If it is hard to touch your toes, you need to improve your suppleness.

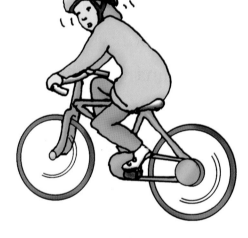

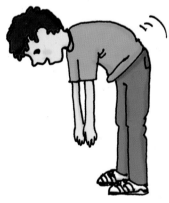

If your legs start to ache when you are cycling, you need to improve your strength.

Swimming can help people of all ages stay fit. The water helps support your body so you do not hurt yourself. Swimming is good for people who are overweight and for people who have disabilities.

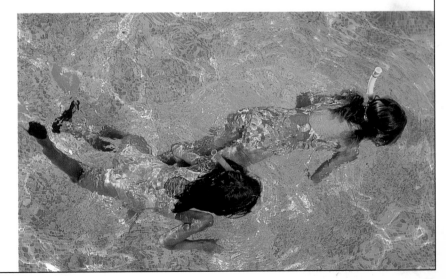

Food for Energy

Food and drink give you energy. When you exercise, you use lots of energy. Each day, you need to eat enough to provide about the same amount of energy that you use.

If you eat too much and do not exercise enough, your body will store the extra energy as fat. If your body stores too much fat, you will be overweight and will be more likely to have health problems. If you do not eat enough, you will lose weight and you will not have enough energy.

Your body needs energy to grow and to work properly even when you are resting. When you are still growing, you need extra energy.

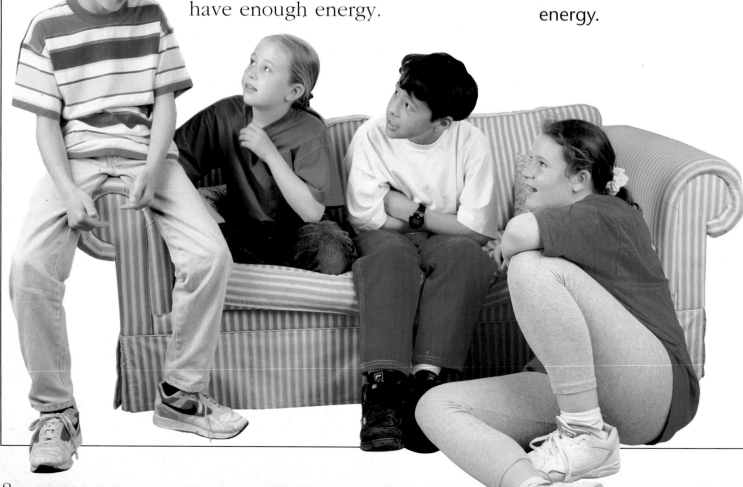

You can find out how much energy is stored in foods by looking at their labels. Energy is measured in calories (cal.). Labels usually show how many calories there are in 3.5 oz. (100 g) of the food. Find out how much energy there is in some of your favorite foods.

To use all the energy from a burger, large fries, and a milk shake, you would need to run for three hours.

A carrot contains 20 cal. of energy.

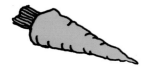

A bowl of breakfast cereal and milk contains 170 cal. of energy.

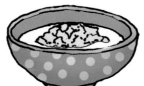

An apple contains 40 cal. of energy.

An egg contains 90 cal. of energy.

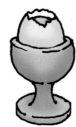

A burger and fries contain 715 cal. of energy.

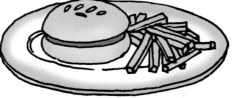

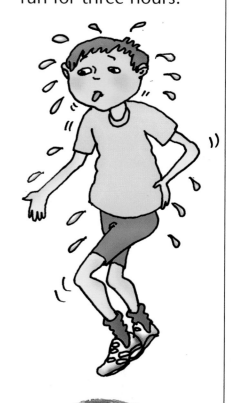

Foods that provide most energy are starchy carbohydrates, which should be the main part of each meal. Your body breaks down carbohydrates into glucose, which it can turn into energy.

Starchy carbohydrates include bread, pasta, potatoes, rice, and cereals.

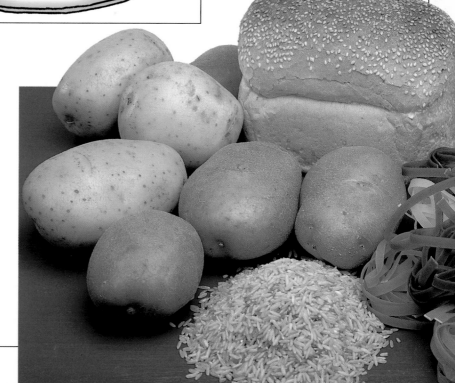

Warming Up and Cooling Down

It is important to warm up and cool down every time you exercise. A warm-up gets your body ready for exercise. It helps your blood carry oxygen to your muscles so they are ready to work. You can warm up by marching or jogging on the spot and doing stretching exercises. Warm up for about five to ten minutes until you feel warm and you are breathing a bit faster than normal.

If your face becomes red when you exercise, it is because blood is rushing to blood vessels near the surface of your skin so the skin can cool itself!

To cool down after exercising, do some slower movements until you are breathing normally again. Cooling down helps keep your muscles from getting stiff and sore.

Stretching after exercise can help you become more supple. Hold each stretch and count to ten.

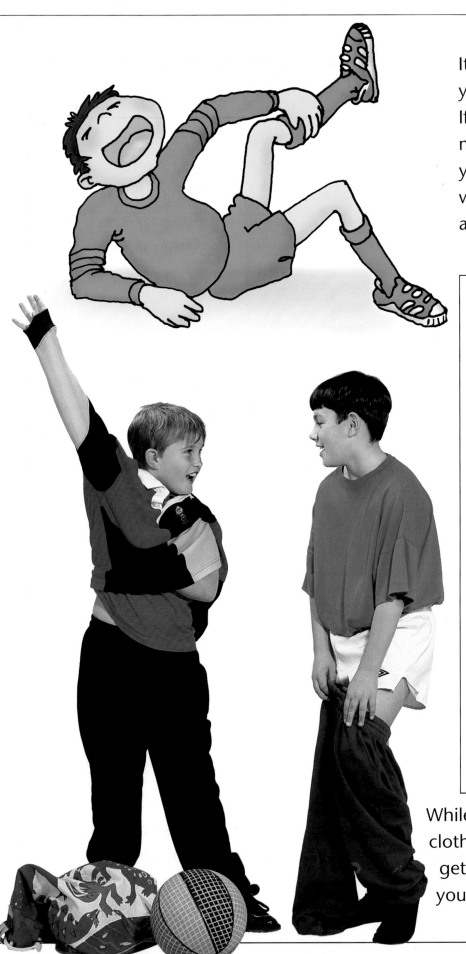

It is important to warm up your muscles before exercising. If you exercise with cold muscles, you might hurt yourself. When muscles are warm, they are more flexible and tear less easily.

Leave a piece of Poster Putty in the refrigerator until it is cold. Try tearing it. Now warm the Poster Putty in your hands. Is it more flexible when it is warm or cold? When does it tear easily?

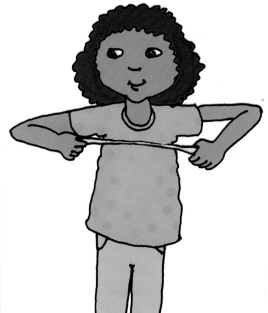

While you cool down, put on warm clothes. Your body will be trying to get rid of the heat it made when you worked your muscles.

Bones and Joints

Your skeleton is your body's framework. It is made up of lots of different bones. Bones give your body its shape and let you stand and move about. Bones are strong and tough and protect the soft parts of your body.

Joints are places where your bones join together, like your knees and elbows. Joints help your body move. Joints are held together by strong straps called ligaments. Shiny cartilage and a special fluid keep the bones from rubbing against each other and from wearing out.

Your body is making new bone cells all the time. Children replace their skeletons about every two years.

Calcium, which comes from milk, dairy foods, and some fruit and vegetables, helps build strong bones.

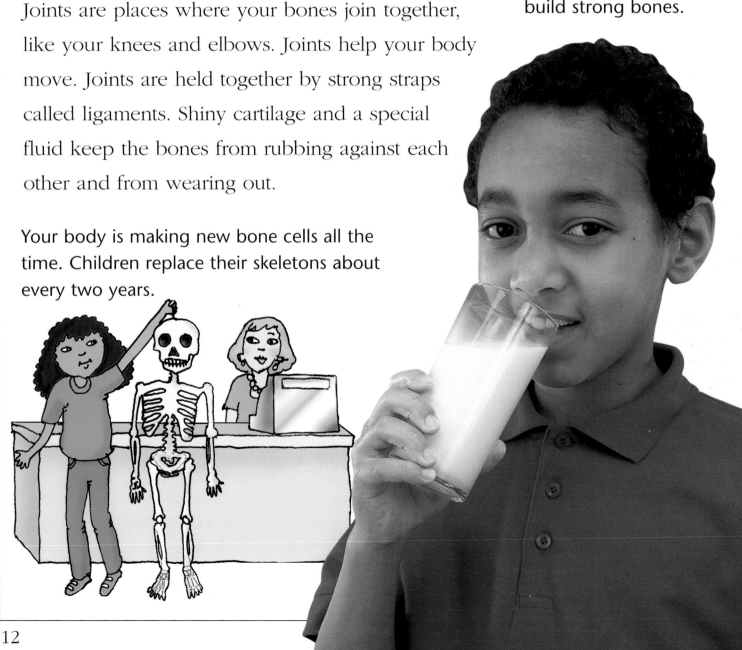

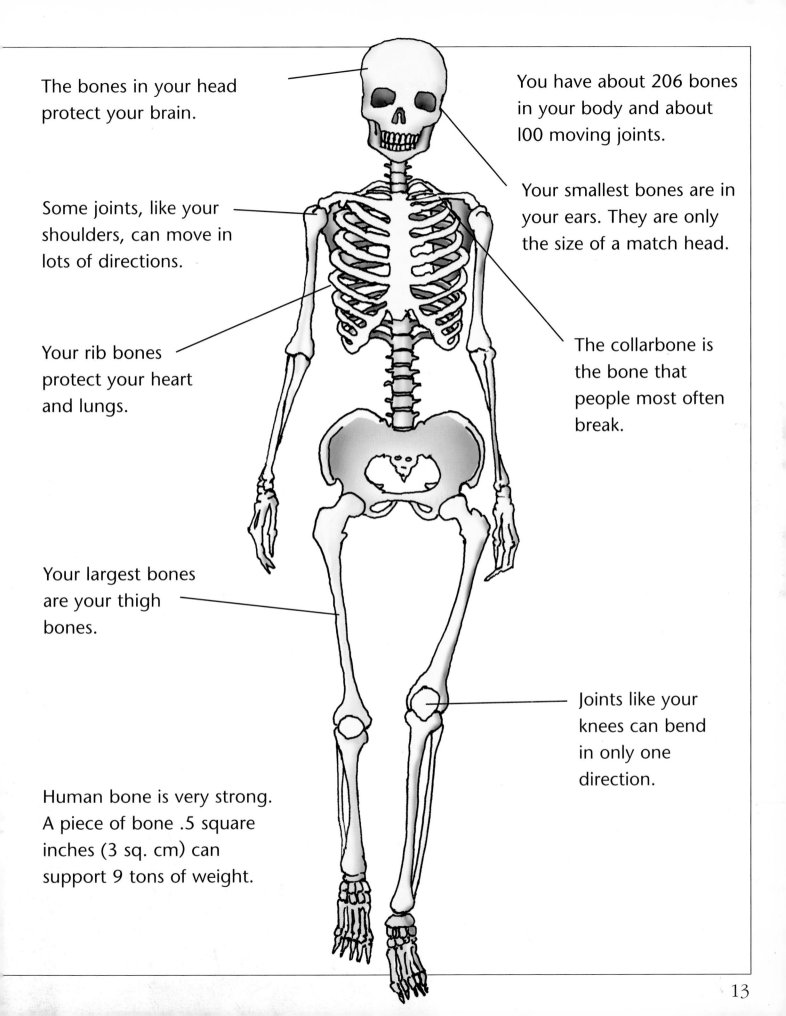

The bones in your head protect your brain.

You have about 206 bones in your body and about 100 moving joints.

Some joints, like your shoulders, can move in lots of directions.

Your smallest bones are in your ears. They are only the size of a match head.

Your rib bones protect your heart and lungs.

The collarbone is the bone that people most often break.

Your largest bones are your thigh bones.

Joints like your knees can bend in only one direction.

Human bone is very strong. A piece of bone .5 square inches (3 sq. cm) can support 9 tons of weight.

13

Exercises for Suppleness

Stretching exercises help keep your joints supple and keep them from getting stiff. Being supple means you can do lots of different movements easily. You can bend, stretch, and twist.

When you exercise, the muscles that work your joints are stretched, so the joints can bend farther. If you do not exercise, your muscles gradually get shorter, and the joints become stiff. As a result you are more likely to hurt yourself when you play sports.

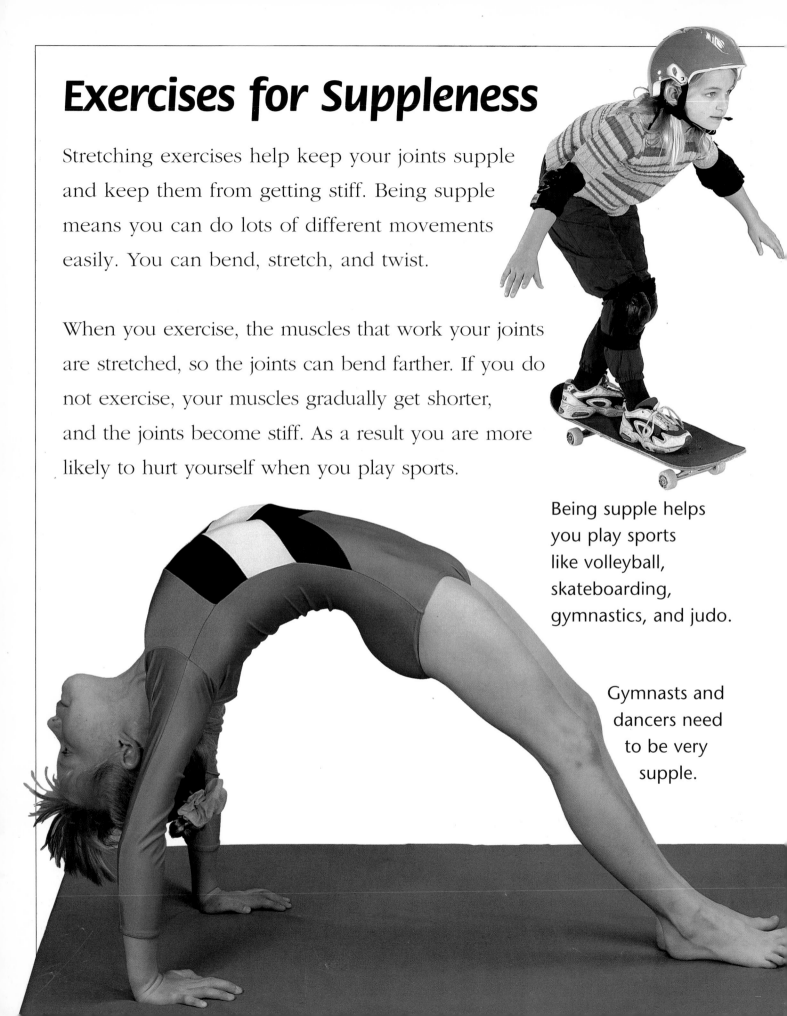

Being supple helps you play sports like volleyball, skateboarding, gymnastics, and judo.

Gymnasts and dancers need to be very supple.

Stretching exercises are good for warming up and cooling down. Try:

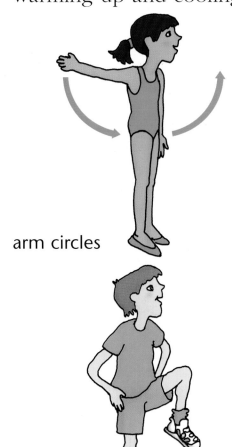

arm circles

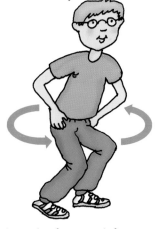

hip circles, with your knees bent

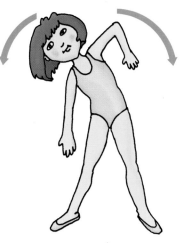

side stretches

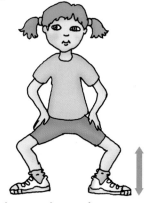

knee lifts

knee bends

Always stretch gently and slowly. Breathe slowly and deeply as you stretch, and hold the stretch for a few seconds.

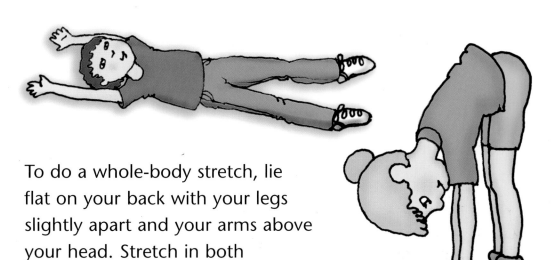

To do a whole-body stretch, lie flat on your back with your legs slightly apart and your arms above your head. Stretch in both directions and count to ten.

When you try touching your toes, you may feel muscles pulling at the backs of your knees. Practice every day, stretching gently, and you will soon find you can bend farther.

Muscles and How They Work

When you exercise, you use your muscles to move your bones. To do this, muscles need energy from food and oxygen from the air. You breathe in air, and oxygen goes into your lungs and then through your blood to your muscles.

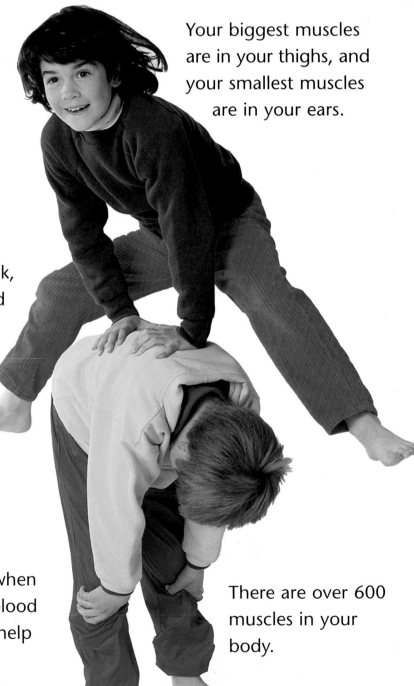

Your biggest muscles are in your thighs, and your smallest muscles are in your ears.

While you exercise, your muscles work harder and need more oxygen. This is why you need to breathe faster when you are active.

You need about 200 muscles to walk, 30 muscles to raise an eyebrow, and 15 muscles to smile.

Using your muscles helps make them stronger.

Some muscles keep working even when you are asleep. Your heart pumps blood around your body, and your lungs help you breathe.

There are over 600 muscles in your body.

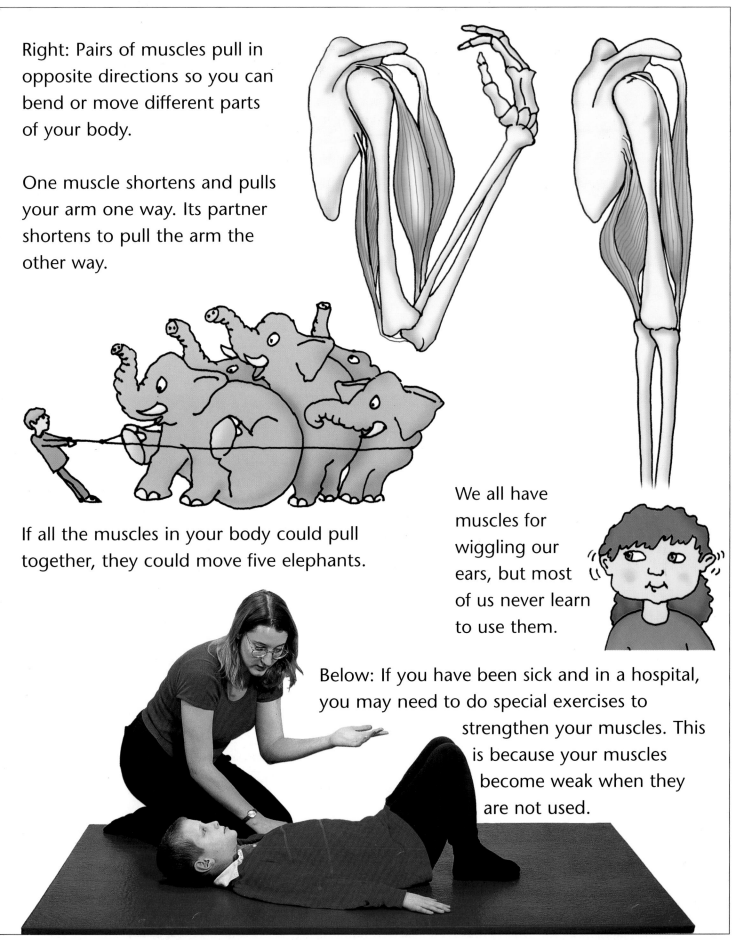

Right: Pairs of muscles pull in opposite directions so you can bend or move different parts of your body.

One muscle shortens and pulls your arm one way. Its partner shortens to pull the arm the other way.

If all the muscles in your body could pull together, they could move five elephants.

We all have muscles for wiggling our ears, but most of us never learn to use them.

Below: If you have been sick and in a hospital, you may need to do special exercises to strengthen your muscles. This is because your muscles become weak when they are not used.

Exercises for Strength

You need to work your muscles to keep them strong. Strong muscles support your joints and help you stand properly. They make it less likely that you will hurt yourself playing sports.

Strong arms help you push, pull, and lift. Strong legs mean you can run, climb, and cycle. Different exercises help different muscles. Swimming is good for all your muscles. Running helps make your leg, back, and shoulder muscles stronger.

Sports like discus throwing build strength in the back, arms, and shoulders.

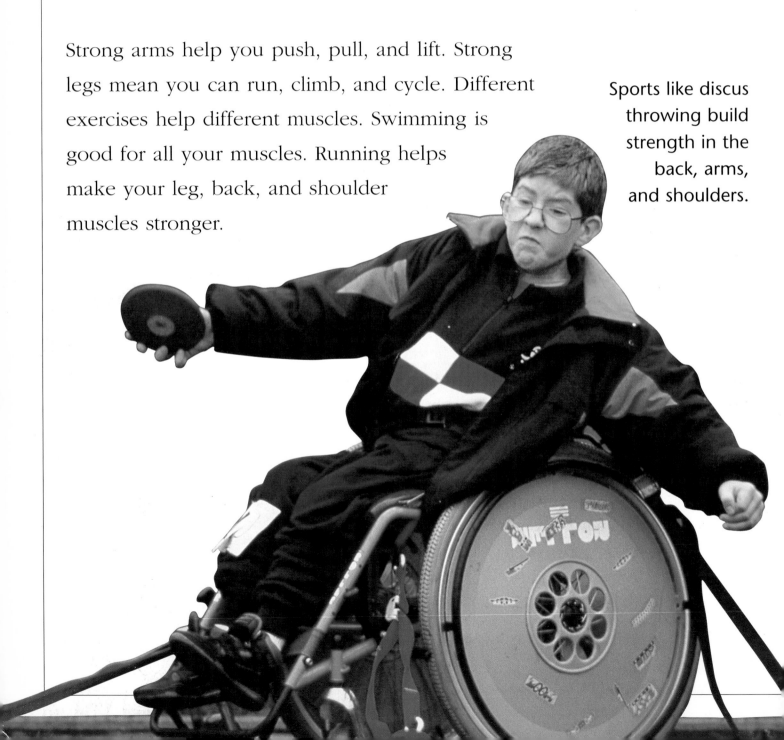

Push-ups make the upper body stronger. Lie on your front with your hands under your shoulders and with your toes pointing to the floor. Push with your arms to lift your body up, keeping your head down and your back straight.

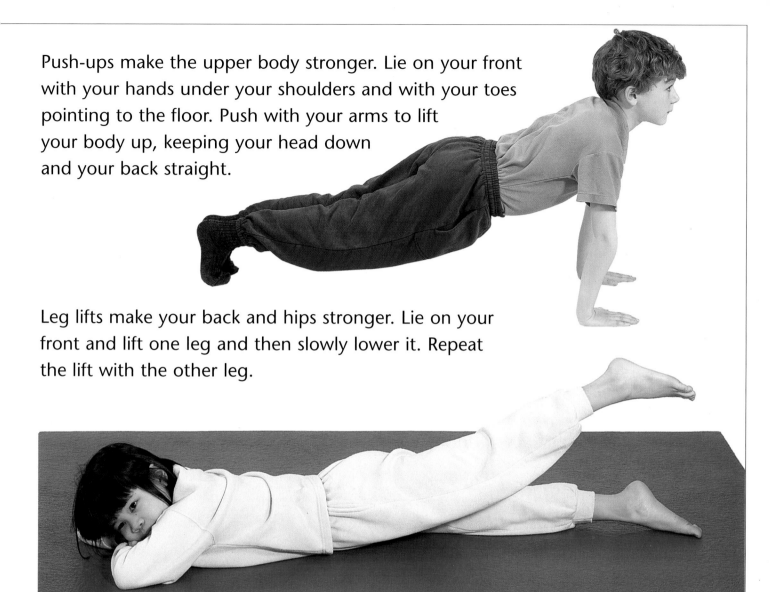

Leg lifts make your back and hips stronger. Lie on your front and lift one leg and then slowly lower it. Repeat the lift with the other leg.

Start by doing these exercises five or six times, until you are strong enough to do more of them easily.

You can even exercise your fingers! Hold a soft rubber ball about 2 in. (5 cm) in diameter in the palm of your hand. Squeeze your fingers around the ball as hard as you can two or three times. Do the same with the other hand.

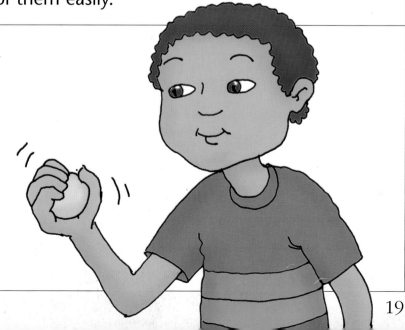

The Heart and Lungs

When you exercise, your heart beats faster and you take faster, deeper breaths. As you breathe in, air goes through your nose and mouth, down a tube into your lungs. Your lungs are like two sacks. They get bigger as they fill with air when you breathe in and smaller when you breathe out.

Oxygen from your lungs goes into your blood and is carried to your muscles. When you exercise, your lungs have to work harder to provide extra oxygen for your muscles.

Blood is pumped around your body by your heart. When you exercise, your heart pumps up to six times more blood than when you are resting.

Exercise makes your heart and lungs stronger.

You take in about 20,000 breaths every day.

Your lungs can hold enough air to fill about 18 soda cans. Breathing deeply doubles the amount of air your lungs hold.

Heart

Heart Facts

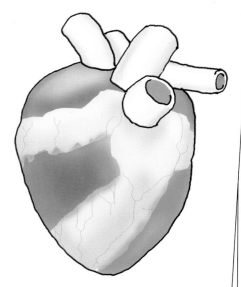

- Your heart beats about 100,000 times a day. It pumps about 16,600 gal. (43,000 l) of blood, enough to fill more than 150 baths.
- Your blood vessels would reach twice around the earth if you stretched them end to end.
- Your heart beats faster when you are nervous, for example, before an exam or a race.
- An adult's heart beats about 70 to 80 times each minute. A canary's heart beats 1,000 times a minute. An elephant's heart beats just 25 times a minute.

You can measure your pulse rate by finding your radial artery. It is under the skin on your wrist, just below your thumb. Place two fingertips over the artery and steady your hand with your thumb under your wrist. Use a stopwatch to count the number of beats in 60 seconds. The result is your resting pulse rate.

Check your pulse rate again, after you have done some exercise. What is the difference?

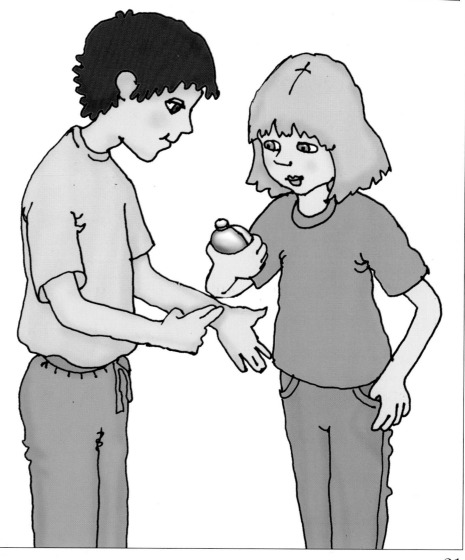

Aerobic Exercise

Aerobic exercise makes your heart and lungs stronger. When you do aerobic exercise, you have to breathe in enough air so that your muscles get enough energy and oxygen to be able to work hard. When you are doing aerobic exercise, you should be breathing faster than usual but not so fast that you cannot talk.

Rollerblading, as well as running, swimming, cycling, dancing, and skipping, all give you aerobic exercise.

Aerobic exercise helps build stamina. As your stamina improves, you will be able to exercise for longer without getting too tired or out of breath.

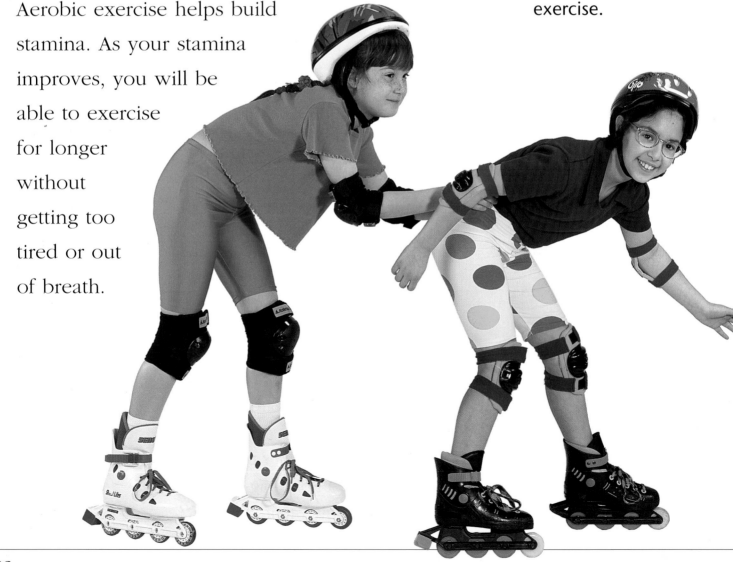

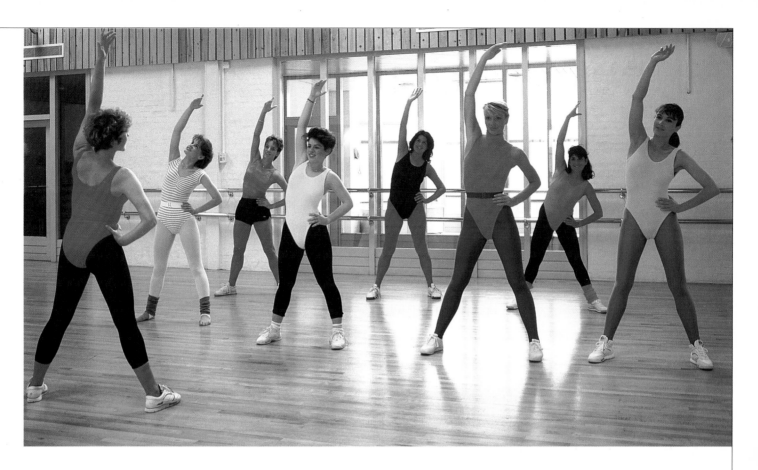

To stay fit, you need to do 20 to 30 minutes of aerobic exercise three times a week, including five minutes to warm up and five minutes to cool down.

Aerobics classes include jumping, jogging, and stretching exercises.

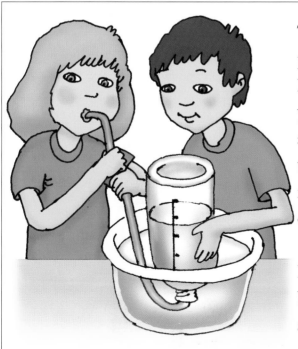

To test your breathing, mark a half-gallon (2-l) plastic bottle in sections of 3.3 fl. oz. (100 ml.). Fill the bottle with water and cover the top with your hand. Then turn the bottle upside down in a bowl half full of water. Get someone to hold the bottle while you feed a plastic tube into the neck. Then try blowing through the other end of the tube as hard as you can.

How much water can you push out of the bottle with one big breath? The air in the bottle shows how much air you had in your lungs.

Exercise Rules

It is important to keep your body safe and comfortable when you are exercising. Do not exercise just after a meal. Your stomach needs blood to help digest your food, so your muscles may not get enough blood to help them work properly. Do not exercise if you are feeling sick or if you have a virus like a cold. Never exercise so hard that your muscles hurt or you feel dizzy, sick, or tired.

If you are getting over an operation or illness or if you have asthma or diabetes, it is best to check with your doctor before exercising or playing sports.

Always drink plenty of water before and during exercise, especially in hot weather. You need to replace the water you lose when you sweat.

Wearing the right clothes for exercise helps keep you safe.

Track suits are good for warming up and cooling down.

Cotton helps keep you cool.

Sports fabrics like lycra are comfortable.

Wear socks to keep your sneakers from rubbing your feet.

Sneakers protect your feet and keep them from getting sore. They must fit properly and have cushioned soles.

Wear layers so that you can take clothes off as your body gets warm. Put on warmer layers after cooling down.

As well as helmets, knee pads, elbow pads, and wrist bands are important for sports like skateboarding and rollerblading.

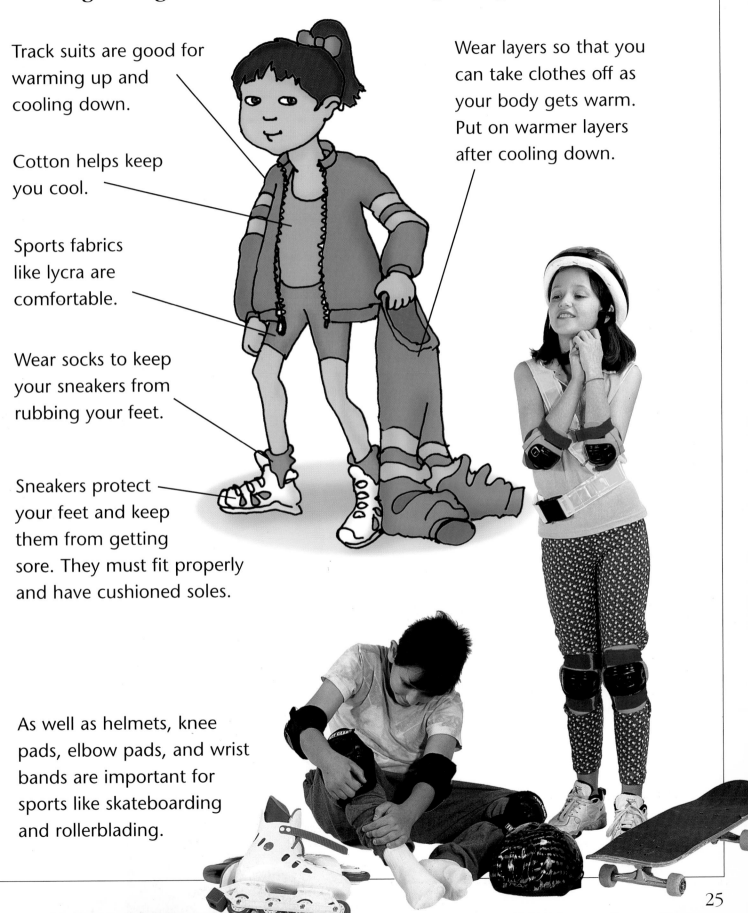

Exercise Plan

Exercise should be part of your daily life. Being active means walking or cycling sometimes rather than going everywhere by car or bus. Climb the stairs instead of taking an elevator.

If you want to stay fit, avoid things that can harm your body, like smoking, taking drugs, and eating too many fatty foods like french fries, cakes, and cookies. Make sure that you eat plenty of fruit and vegetables.

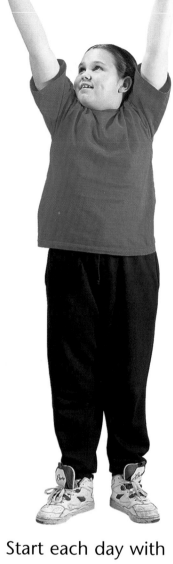

Start each day with a few minutes of stretching.

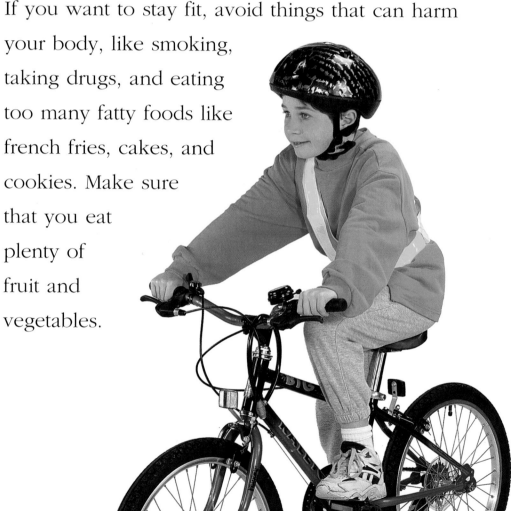

As well as doing things like watching television and using computers, make sure you get some exercise in the fresh air every day.

Rest is important for keeping fit. Sleep is your body's way of getting rest and repairing itself. Children need more sleep than adults do.

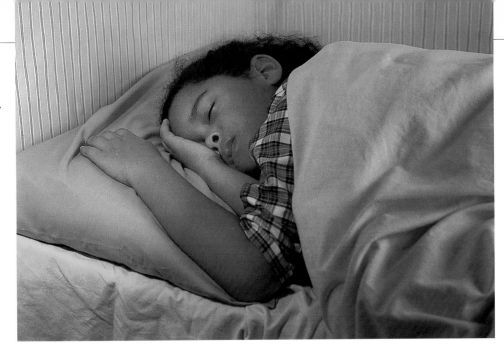

Draw up your own fitness program.

Choose activities you enjoy and make a chart to show when you will do them each week. Leave boxes to check off when you complete each activity.

Try to include:

3 days a week:
5 minutes warmup
20 minutes aerobic exercise
5 minutes cooldown

2 days a week:
15 minutes stretching exercises
15 minutes strength exercises
5 minutes cooldown

1 day a week:
30 minutes of games or sports.

Don't forget to do some stretching every day!

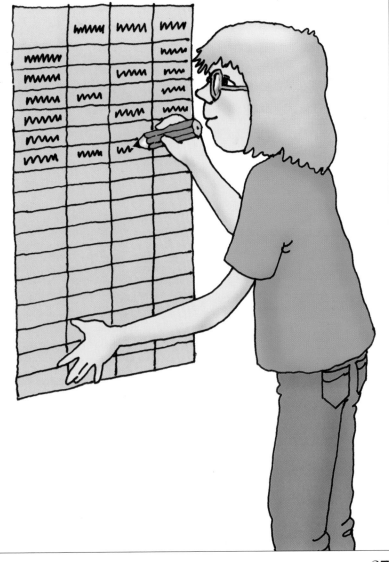

Exercise Is Fun!

You can make new friends by exercising with others. Check out the activities at your local sports club or ask for information at the library. There may be classes in activities like aerobics, swimming, judo, karate, and gymnastics and team sports like soccer and volleyball. It is important to choose activities that you enjoy. Most sports clubs have courts or fields and equipment you can rent.

Joining team games like soccer, volleyball, and basketball is a good way of making friends.

Try to get your family or friends to exercise with you. It is more fun if you exercise together.

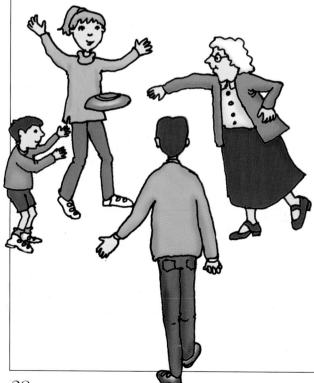

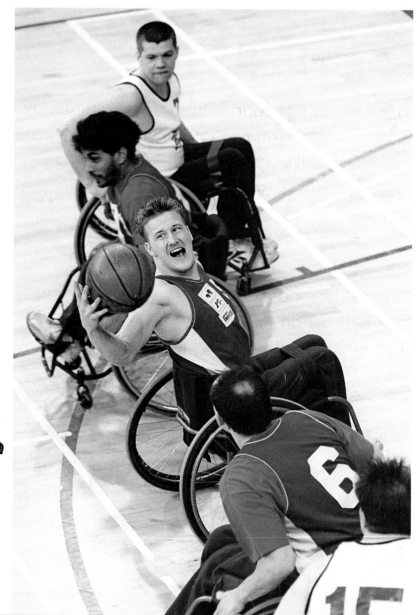

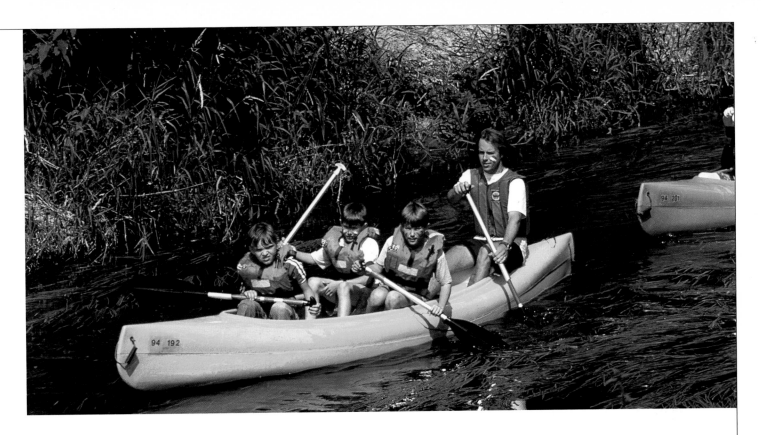

There are lots of sports clubs that organize day trips and vacations. You can choose from many activities, including walking, swimming, tennis, and cycling. You can also learn new skills like canoeing, windsurfing, and climbing.

Walking is good exercise, as well as being fun. And it costs nothing!

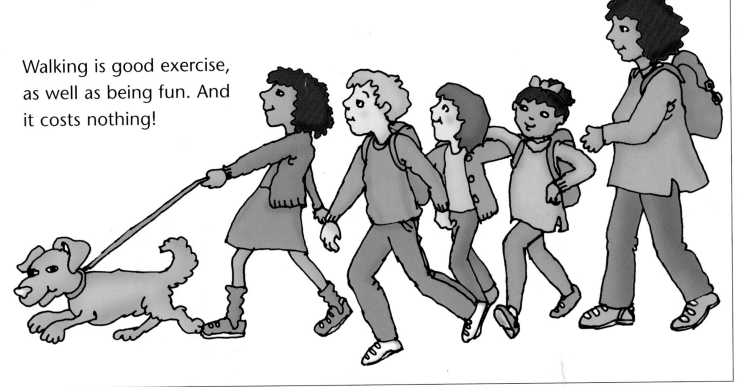

Glossary

Aerobic A type of exercise that uses lots of oxygen from the air and makes the heart and lungs stronger.

Artery A blood vessel that carries blood away from the heart.

Asthma Problems with breathing.

Blood vessels Tubes that carry blood around your body.

Calories Measurements of the energy in food.

Carbohydrates Starchy or sugary foods that give you energy.

Diabetes A disease that means the body cannot control the amount of sugar glucose in the blood.

Digest The way in which the body breaks down food and uses it.

Stamina The ability to keep exercising without getting too tired or out of breath.

Suppleness Being able to move freely and easily.

Virus A type of disease.

Books to Read

Nardo, Don. *Exercise* (Healthy Body.) New York: Chelsea House, 1992.

Reef, Catherine. *Stay Fit: Build a Strong Body* (Good Health Guidelines.) New York: 21st Century Books, 1993.

Savage, Jeff. *Aerobics* (Working Out.) Parsippany, NJ: Crestwood House, 1995.

Schwarzenegger, Arnold & Chas. Gaines. *Arnold's Fitness for Kids Age Birth to Five: A Guide to Health, Exercise, and Nutrition*. New York: Doubleday, 1993.

Index